TIMELESS LONGEVITY

THE SCIENCE OF STAYING YOUNG AND VIBRANT

The Quest For Eternal Youth

By

Dr. Elvira S. Graves

TABLE OF CONTENTS

1. TABLE OF CONTENTS
2. Disclaimer
3. Introduction
4. Chapter 1: The Biology of Aging
5. Chapter 2: The Psychology of Aging
6. Chapter 3: Social Dimensions of Aging
7. Chapter 4: Nutrition and Longevity
8. Chapter 5: Physical Activity and Aging
9. Chapter 6: Technological Advances in Aging
10. Chapter 7: Personal Stories of Longevity
11. Conclusion

Dedication

To my late dad who wishes to long enough to see me succeed in my career as he always wanted for all his children.

Disclaimer

Copyright © by Dr. Elvira S. Graves 2024.
All rights reserved.
Before this document is duplicated or reproduced in any manner, the publisher's consent must be gained. Therefore, the contents within can neither be stored electronically, transferred, nor kept in a database. Neither in Part nor full can the document be copied, scanned, faxed, or retained without approval from the publisher or creator.

Introduction

The Quest for Eternal Youth: Exploring the Human Fascination with Staying Young
In a world obsessed with youth and beauty, the quest for eternal youth has become a timeless pursuit. From ancient civilizations to modern society, the desire to defy the aging process and maintain a youthful appearance has captivated the human imagination. But what drives this fascination with staying young, and is eternal youth truly attainable? Apart from the quest to live and achieve your purpose and mission, we also do not want to leave our loved ones behind seeing the good times and memories we keep having daily. Man as an animal wishes to live long enough if not forever, especially with the recent development in technology that has made

our lives super easy and enjoyable more than ever in human history. There's always a quest as to whether one can have a medicine that will buy life or extend it to another century.

I strongly believe every day scientists are constantly researching to answer this question. But before then you can take care of your health and live meaningful and well long enough to accomplish all you ever wish to. One important thing you must keep at the back of your mind is that life is not about how long you live but how well and the impact you have in the life of humanity that matters. **"LIFE IS NOT MEASURED BY DURATION BUT BY DONATION"**.

The Fascination with Eternal Youth
Throughout history, cultures have revered youth for its vitality, beauty, and potential. The concept of eternal youth is deeply rooted in mythology, folklore, and literature, where tales

of fountains of youth and immortal beings have captured our

collective imagination. In today's world, the media plays a significant role in perpetuating the idea that youth equates to success, happiness, and desirability. Advertisements, movies, and social media platforms often promote youth-centric ideals, creating pressure to defy the natural process of aging. But that's not the complete truth. There's so much you can do as you age. Usefulness and youthfulness are the state of the mind. If your mind is young, you will achieve whatever you set your mind on. Your main job now is to take care of your body now so that it will take care of you later. Your body and you operate in a reverse way, meaning; what your body requires to live long doesn't make sense to you, while what you are craving doesn't make sense to your body at all. If you can learn to balance this, congratulations.

Defining Aging

Aging is a complex phenomenon influenced by a combination of biological, psychological, and social factors. At the biological level, aging is

characterized by a gradual decline in cellular function, leading to changes in physical appearance and health. It also affects the level of your operation when it comes to stamina and physique. Psychologically, aging can bring about feelings of loss, identity shifts, and existential contemplation. It also rundowns the capacity of your mental health and changes the overall dynamics of how you behave. Socially, aging is often associated with stereotypes, discrimination, and marginalization, highlighting the need for a more inclusive and age-friendly society.
The focal point is that, there's a retardation In your overall performance and expectations generally.

The Science of Longevity
Advances in medical research have shed light on the mechanisms of aging and potential strategies

for extending lifespan. From genetic studies to lifestyle interventions, scientists are uncovering the secrets to longevity. Factors such as diet,

exercise, stress management, and social connections have been identified as key influencers of aging processes. While genetics play a role in determining our predisposition to age-related diseases, lifestyle choices can significantly impact how we age.

Embracing Aging
As we navigate the journey of aging, it is essential to shift our perspectives and embrace the process with grace and acceptance. Finding beauty and wisdom in growing old can lead to a more fulfilling and enriching life experience. By adopting healthy habits, cultivating meaningful relationships, and staying mentally engaged, we can enhance our quality of life as we age.

Myths and Misconceptions
There are many myths and misconceptions surrounding aging, from the belief that wrinkles

are inevitable to the notion that old age equates to frailty and dependence. By challenging these stereotypes and reframing our understanding of

aging, we can create a more positive and empowering narrative around growing old. Aging is not a decline but a transformation, offering new opportunities for growth and self-discovery.

Cultural Differences in Aging
Attitudes towards aging vary across cultures, with some societies revering the wisdom and experience of older individuals, while others prioritize youth and productivity. Cultural beliefs and traditions shape our perceptions of aging and influence how we approach the process of growing old. By exploring different cultural perspectives on longevity, we can gain a deeper appreciation for the diversity of aging experiences worldwide.

The Emotional Journey

Coping with the emotional aspects of aging can be a challenging yet rewarding process. From facing the fear of mortality to embracing the changes that come with growing old, navigating

the emotional terrain of aging requires resilience and self-awareness. By finding joy in the present moment, cultivating gratitude for life's blessings, and accepting the inevitability of change, we can approach aging with a sense of peace and acceptance.

Nutrition and Longevity
The food we eat plays a crucial role in promoting longevity and overall well-being. A diet rich in fruits, vegetables, whole grains, and lean proteins can provide essential nutrients and antioxidants that support healthy aging. Superfoods such as blueberries, kale, and salmon are known for their anti-aging properties, helping to combat inflammation, oxidative stress, and age-related diseases. Staying hydrated and maintaining a balanced diet are key pillars of healthy aging.

Exercise and Longevity
Physical activity is another cornerstone of healthy aging, offering a myriad of benefits for

both body and mind. Regular exercise can improve cardiovascular health, strengthen muscles and bones, and enhance cognitive function. From yoga and tai chi to strength training and aerobic exercises, there are numerous ways to stay active and mobile as we age. Incorporating movement into our daily routines can help us maintain independence, vitality, and a sense of well-being.

Mental Well-being
Caring for our mental health is essential for successful aging and longevity. Engaging in activities that stimulate the mind, such as reading, puzzles, and learning new skills, can help preserve cognitive function and prevent age-related cognitive decline. Practicing mindfulness, meditation, and stress management techniques can promote emotional resilience and

psychological well-being. By prioritizing mental wellness, we can cultivate a positive outlook on aging and navigate life's challenges with grace and equanimity.

Social Connections
Maintaining strong social connections is vital for healthy aging and longevity. Building a support network of friends, family, and community members can provide emotional support, companionship, and a sense of belonging. Combating loneliness and isolation is crucial for overall well-being, as social interactions can boost mood, reduce stress, and enhance quality of life. By staying connected to others and engaging in meaningful relationships, we can age gracefully and joyfully.

Medical Advances in Aging
The field of anti-aging medicine is rapidly evolving, with breakthroughs and innovations offering promising prospects for extending lifespan and improving health outcomes in old age. From regenerative therapies to personalized

medicine, researchers are exploring cutting-edge approaches to age-related diseases and age reversal. Ethical considerations surrounding longevity research, such as access to treatments

and the implications of life extension, are also being debated within the scientific community. As we navigate the frontiers of medical science, it is essential to consider the ethical, social, and philosophical implications of extending human lifespan.

In conclusion, the quest for eternal youth is a multifaceted journey that encompasses biological, psychological, social, and cultural dimensions. By redefining our understanding of aging, embracing the process with grace and acceptance, and adopting healthy lifestyle habits, we can enhance our quality of life and promote longevity. As we navigate the complexities of growing old in a youth-centric society, it is essential to cultivate a positive mindset, prioritize self-care, and nurture meaningful connections with others. Aging is not a curse but a privilege, offering us the opportunity to evolve, learn, and grow in wisdom and grace. Embrace the journey of aging with an open heart and a

resilient spirit, and let the beauty of each passing year illuminate your path towards a fulfilling and purposeful life.

Chapter 1: The Biology of Aging

As we delve into the intricate processes that govern aging, it is essential to explore the underlying biological mechanisms that drive this natural phenomenon. From the ticking of cellular clocks to the influence of our genetic blueprint, and the internal factors that accelerate aging, understanding the biology of aging is key to unlocking the secrets of longevity and healthy aging.

Cellular Clocks: Telomeres and Cellular Aging

At the heart of cellular aging lies the concept of telomeres, the protective caps at the end of our chromosomes that safeguard our genetic material. Telomeres act as cellular clocks, gradually shortening with each cell division until they reach a critical length, signaling cell senescence or death. This process, known as replicative senescence, plays a crucial role in the aging of our cells and tissues.

Telomeres are composed of repetitive DNA sequences and associated proteins that prevent the loss of essential genetic information during cell division. As cells replicate, telomeres shorten, eventually leading to cellular dysfunction and senescence. Shortened telomeres are associated with age-related diseases, such as cardiovascular disorders, cancer, and neurodegenerative conditions.

To maintain telomere length and promote healthy aging, various lifestyle factors can play a significant role. Adequate sleep, stress

Management, regular exercise, and a balanced diet rich in antioxidants and nutrients can support telomere maintenance and cellular health. Additionally, practices such as meditation, mindfulness, and social connections have been linked to telomere preservation and longevity.

The Role of Genetics in Longevity
Our genetic makeup plays a significant role in determining our lifespan and susceptibility to age-related diseases. While genetics alone do not dictate our fate, they can influence how we age and our predisposition to certain health conditions. Longevity genes, such as FOXO3, APOE, and SIRT1, have been identified as key players in regulating aging processes and promoting longevity.

Genetic variations in these longevity genes can impact cellular pathways involved in DNA repair, inflammation, and oxidative stress, influencing how our bodies respond to aging.

For example, individuals with a specific variant of the FOXO3 gene have been found to have a higher likelihood of living to an advanced age. Similarly, the APOE gene is associated with the risk of developing Alzheimer's disease and cardiovascular disorders. By understanding our genetic profile and potential risk factors for age-related conditions, we can proactively mitigate these risks and promote healthy aging. Genetic testing and personalized medicine offer insights into our genetic predispositions, allowing for tailored interventions and lifestyle modifications to optimize health and longevity.

Oxidative Stress and Inflammation in Aging
Oxidative stress and inflammation are internal factors contributing to aging, accelerating cellular damage and tissue degeneration. Oxidative stress occurs when an imbalance between free radicals and antioxidants in the body leads to oxidative damage to proteins, lipids, and DNA. This process can impair

cellular function and contribute to age-related diseases.

Factors that contribute to oxidative stress include environmental toxins, poor diet, smoking, and chronic stress. By reducing exposure to oxidative stressors and increasing antioxidant intake through a diet rich in fruits, vegetables, and whole grains, we can mitigate the harmful effects of oxidative stress and support healthy aging.
Several factors contribute to oxidative stress, with environmental toxins, poor diet, smoking, and chronic stress being significant culprits:

Environmental Toxins: Exposure to environmental pollutants, such as air pollution, heavy metals, pesticides, and industrial chemicals, can increase oxidative stress in the body. These toxins generate free radicals and reactive oxygen species, leading to oxidative damage to cells and tissues. Long-term exposure to environmental toxins can contribute to the development of various health conditions, including cardiovascular disease, respiratory disorders, and cancer.

Poor Diet: A diet high in processed foods, refined sugars, trans fats, and artificial additives can promote oxidative stress in the body. These unhealthy dietary choices lack essential nutrients and antioxidants that help combat free radicals and support cellular health. Inadequate intake of fruits, vegetables, whole grains, and lean proteins deprives the body of vital antioxidants, making it more susceptible to oxidative damage and age-related diseases.

Smoking: Cigarette smoke contains a plethora of harmful chemicals and free radicals that induce oxidative stress in the body. The toxic compounds in tobacco smoke trigger an inflammatory response and generate oxidative damage to cells and tissues. Chronic smoking not only depletes the body's antioxidant defenses but also impairs cellular function and accelerates the aging process. Smoking is a major risk factor for various health conditions, including lung cancer, heart disease, and respiratory disorders, largely due to its pro-oxidant effects.

Chronic Stress: Prolonged exposure to psychological stress can increase oxidative stress levels in the body and disrupt cellular homeostasis. Stress triggers the release of stress hormones, such as cortisol and adrenaline, which can promote the production of free radicals and inflammatory mediators. Chronic stress impairs the body's ability to regulate oxidative balance, leading to oxidative damage and systemic inflammation. Over time, chronic stress can contribute to the development of stress-related disorders, mental health issues, and chronic diseases.

Inflammation is another key player in the aging process, with chronic low-grade inflammation contributing to the development of age-related conditions such as arthritis, cardiovascular disease, and neurodegenerative disorders.

Inflammatory cytokines and immune responses can disrupt cellular function and tissue homeostasis, leading to accelerated aging and disease progression.

To combat inflammation and promote healthy aging, lifestyle interventions such as regular exercise, stress management, and an anti-inflammatory diet can be beneficial. Incorporating omega-3 fatty acids, turmeric, and green tea into our diet can help reduce inflammation and support immune function. By addressing oxidative stress and inflammation through holistic approaches, we can enhance our resilience to aging and optimize our well-being as we grow older.

In conclusion, the biology of aging is a complex interplay of cellular processes, genetic influences, and internal factors that shape how we age and our susceptibility to age-related diseases. By understanding the mechanisms of cellular aging, the role of genetics in longevity, and the impact of oxidative stress and inflammation on aging, we can take proactive steps to promote healthy aging and enhance our quality of life as we journey through the golden years. Embracing the science of aging with curiosity and resilience, we can unlock the secrets of longevity and age gracefully with vitality and purpose.

Chapter 2: The Psychology of Aging

As we journey through the later stages of life, the psychological aspects of aging come to the forefront, shaping our perceptions, memories, cognition, and emotional well-being. Understanding how aging influences our experience of time, memory, and emotions is essential for navigating the complexities of growing old with grace and resilience.

Perception of Time: Aging and the Experience of Life's Passage

One of the profound ways in which aging impacts our psychology is through the shifting perception of time. As we grow older, time may seem to pass more quickly, with years blending into one another and life milestones becoming more significant. Reflecting on the passage of time can evoke a range of emotions, from nostalgia to anticipation for the future.

For example, an individual approaching retirement may feel a mix of excitement and apprehension about the next chapter of their life. Memories of past achievements and experiences may take on new meaning as they contemplate the legacy they wish to leave behind. Embracing the passage of time with grace and acceptance involves acknowledging the inevitability of change and finding meaning in each moment.

Strategies for enhancing the perception of time in later years include mindfulness practices, journaling, and engaging in activities that bring joy and fulfillment. By savoring the present moment, cultivating gratitude for life's blessings, and cherishing relationships with loved ones, individuals can enrich their experience of time and find peace in the ebb and flow of life's rhythms.

Memory and Cognition in Aging
Maintaining mental acuity and memory function is a vital aspect of healthy aging. While cognitive changes are a natural part of the aging process, there are ways to support brain health and preserve cognitive function as we grow older. Engaging in activities that stimulate the mind, such as puzzles, reading, and learning new skills, can help keep the brain sharp and agile.

For example, a retiree who takes up painting as a hobby not only enhances their creativity but also boosts their cognitive abilities through visual-spatial processing and problem-solving. By challenging the brain with novel experiences and intellectual pursuits, individuals can build cognitive reserve and reduce the risk of cognitive decline in later life.

The importance of cognitive stimulation and brain health in aging cannot be overstated. Regular physical exercise, a balanced diet rich in brain-boosting nutrients, and social engagement are key pillars of cognitive well-being. By prioritizing brain health and mental acuity, individuals can maintain their cognitive vitality and independence as they age.

Emotional Resilience and Well-being
Cultivating emotional resilience and well-being in later life is essential for navigating the inevitable challenges and transitions that come with aging. From coping with loss and grief to finding joy and purpose in everyday moments, emotional resilience enables individuals to adapt to life's changes with grace and positivity.

For example, an older adult who loses a spouse may experience profound grief and loneliness but finds solace in connecting with friends, pursuing hobbies, and seeking support from a therapist or support group. By acknowledging their emotions, expressing their feelings, and engaging in self-care practices, they can cultivate emotional resilience and navigate the grieving process with courage and strength.

Examples of emotional resilience in later life include finding meaning and purpose in volunteer work, maintaining a sense of humor and optimism in the face of adversity, and fostering deep connections with others. By embracing the full spectrum of human emotions and experiences, individuals can cultivate happiness and well-being in their later years, enriching their lives and those around them.

In conclusion, the psychology of aging encompasses a rich tapestry of perceptions, memories, cognition, and emotions that shape our experience of growing old. By embracing the passage of time with grace, maintaining mental acuity and memory function, and cultivating emotional resilience and well-being, individuals can navigate the complexities of aging with resilience and vitality. Embracing the psychological aspects of aging with curiosity and compassion, we can unlock the secrets to a fulfilling and purposeful life in the golden years.

Chapter 3: Social Dimensions of Aging

Cultural Attitudes: How Different Societies View Aging

Cultural attitudes towards aging play a significant role in shaping the experiences and perceptions of older adults within different societies. These attitudes are deeply rooted in the values, beliefs, and traditions of a culture, influencing how aging is viewed, respected, and integrated into the fabric of society. By examining how various cultures approach aging, we can gain insights into the diverse ways in which older individuals are valued and respected across the world.

In Japan, older individuals are held in high esteem for their wisdom, experience, and contributions to society. The concept of filial piety, which emphasizes respect for one's elders and ancestors, is deeply ingrained in Japanese culture. Older adults are revered for their knowledge, guidance, and moral authority, with a strong emphasis on maintaining close family ties and honoring the wisdom of previous generations. In Japanese society, aging is often associated with dignity, honor, and a sense of duty towards one's family and community.

Conversely, in Western cultures, there is often a youth-centric focus that can lead to ageism and stereotypes about aging. The emphasis on youthfulness, productivity, and physical appearance in Western societies can marginalize older adults and perpetuate negative stereotypes about aging. Older individuals may face discrimination in the workplace, healthcare settings, and media portrayals, contributing to feelings of invisibility, isolation, and devaluation. The societal pressure to remain youthful and productive can create barriers for older adults seeking to actively participate and contribute to society.

In Indigenous communities, elders hold a central role in decision-making, governance, and passing down traditional knowledge to younger generations. Elders are respected as the bearers of cultural heritage, oral traditions, and spiritual wisdom, serving as mentors and guides for the community. The intergenerational exchange of knowledge and values is highly valued in Indigenous cultures, with elders playing a vital role in preserving cultural identity and promoting social cohesion. The wisdom and experience of elders are honored and celebrated, fostering a deep sense of respect, reciprocity, and interconnectedness within the community.

Overall, cultural attitudes towards aging reflect broader societal values, norms, and intergenerational dynamics within a given culture. By recognizing and appreciating the diverse ways in which different societies view and honor older adults, we can gain a deeper understanding of the complexities of aging and the importance of valuing the wisdom, experience, and contributions of older individuals across cultures. Embracing a more inclusive and age-friendly approach to aging can help combat ageism, foster intergenerational connections, and create a more equitable and compassionate society for individuals of all ages.

The Wisdom of Experience: Valuing the Contributions of the Elderly
The wisdom and experience of older adults are highly valued for the invaluable contributions they bring to communities and society as a whole. By recognizing and honoring the wisdom of older individuals, we can tap into a wealth of knowledge, foster intergenerational connections, and create a more inclusive and age-friendly society.

Tapping into a Wealth of Knowledge and Life Lessons: Older adults have accumulated a lifetime of experiences, insights, and wisdom that can serve as a valuable resource for guiding younger generations. Their stories, lessons learned, and perspectives on life can offer invaluable guidance, mentorship, and inspiration to individuals of all ages. By tapping into this wealth of knowledge, younger generations can benefit from the wisdom and expertise of older adults, gaining a deeper understanding of history, culture, and human experience.

Fostering Intergenerational Connections and Mutual Respect: Valuing the contributions of the elderly fosters intergenerational connections and mutual respect between individuals of different age groups. By creating opportunities for meaningful interactions and dialogue between older and younger generations, we can bridge generational divides, promote empathy, and cultivate a sense of shared humanity. Intergenerational relationships can enrich the lives of both older and younger individuals, fostering a sense of belonging, understanding, and respect across age boundaries.

Creating a More Inclusive and Age-Friendly Society: Recognizing and honoring the wisdom and experience of older adults is essential for creating a more inclusive and age-friendly society. By valuing the contributions of the elderly, we can challenge ageist attitudes, promote diversity, and create environments that respect and support individuals of all ages. An age-friendly society values the unique perspectives, talents, and contributions of older adults, fostering a culture of respect, dignity, and inclusion for individuals at every stage of life.

Building Community: The Importance of Social Connections in Promoting Longevity Building community through social connections is essential for promoting longevity and overall well-being in older adults. By fostering strong social connections, individuals can experience emotional support, enhance their mental and physical health, and cultivate a sense of belonging and purpose within a supportive network.

1. Providing Emotional Support and Companionship: Social connections offer emotional support and companionship, reducing feelings of loneliness and isolation that can negatively impact mental health and well-being. By maintaining close relationships with family, friends, and community members, older adults can share their joys and sorrows, seek comfort during challenging times, and feel a sense of connection and belonging. Emotional support from social connections can provide a source of strength, resilience, and comfort, promoting mental wellness and reducing feelings of loneliness and isolation.

2. Enhancing Mental and Physical Health through Social Engagement: Social engagement and interaction have been linked to improved mental and physical health outcomes in older adults. By participating in social activities, group gatherings, and community events, individuals can stay mentally stimulated, emotionally engaged, and physically active. Social connections can provide opportunities for cognitive stimulation, emotional expression, and physical exercise, contributing to overall well-being and quality of life. Regular social engagement has been associated with reduced stress levels, improved mood, and enhanced cognitive function, promoting mental and physical health in older adults.

3. Creating a Sense of Belonging and Purpose, Fostering a Strong Support Network: Social connections create a sense of belonging and purpose, fostering a strong support network that individuals can rely on in times of need. By cultivating meaningful relationships and building a supportive community, older adults can feel valued, respected, and connected to others. A sense of belonging and purpose can provide motivation, inspiration, and a sense of fulfillment, enhancing overall well-being and quality of life. Having a strong support network of friends, family, and community members can offer practical assistance, emotional encouragement, and a sense of security, promoting resilience and longevity in older adults.

In conclusion, building community through social connections is vital for promoting longevity, well-being, and quality of life in older adults. By nurturing social connections, individuals can access emotional support, enhance their mental and physical health, and cultivate a sense of belonging and purpose within a supportive network. Strong social connections contribute to resilience, happiness, and overall well-being, creating a foundation for healthy aging and fulfilling life in later years. Embracing the importance of social connections in promoting longevity can lead to a more vibrant, connected, and supportive community where individuals of all ages thrive and flourish together.

Chapter 4: Nutrition and Longevity

Eating well is not just about satisfying hunger; it is about fueling our bodies with the nutrients they need to thrive and flourish. In this chapter, we will explore the science of nutrition and its impact on longevity, discover superfoods that can support healthy aging, and debunk common myths surrounding dieting and nutrition.

The Science of Eating Well: Nutritional Strategies to Slow Aging
Nutrition plays a crucial role in the aging process, influencing our overall health and well-being. By adopting healthy eating habits and making informed food choices, we can slow down the aging process and promote longevity.

Nutritional strategies to support healthy aging include:

- **Balanced Diet**: Consuming a balanced diet rich in fruits, vegetables, whole grains, lean proteins, and healthy fats provides essential nutrients that support cellular function, immune health, and overall vitality.

- **Hydration**: Staying hydrated is key to maintaining optimal bodily functions, supporting digestion, circulation, and nutrient absorption. Drinking an adequate amount of water throughout the day is essential for overall health and well-being.

- **Portion Control**: Monitoring portion sizes and practicing mindful eating can help prevent overeating and promote healthy weight management. Portion control is essential for maintaining a balanced and nutritious diet.

By incorporating these nutritional strategies into our daily routine, we can nourish our bodies, support healthy aging, and enhance our quality of life as we grow older.

Superfoods for Seniors: Best Foods for Maintaining Youth and Vitality
Certain foods are packed with nutrients that can support healthy aging and vitality. These superfoods are rich in antioxidants, vitamins, minerals, and other beneficial compounds that promote overall well-being. Some of the best superfoods for seniors include:

1. Blueberries: Rich in antioxidants, blueberries can help reduce inflammation, improve cognitive function, and support heart health.

2. Salmon: A great source of omega-3 fatty acids, salmon can support brain health, reduce inflammation, and promote cardiovascular health.

3. Spinach: Packed with vitamins, minerals, and antioxidants, spinach can support bone health, eye health, and immune function.

4. Nuts and Seeds: Almonds, walnuts, chia seeds, and flax seeds are rich in healthy fats, fiber, and protein, supporting heart health, brain function, and overall well-being.

By incorporating these superfoods into their diet, seniors can nourish their bodies, support healthy aging, and enhance their vitality and quality of life.

The Myths and Realities of Dieting: Separating Fact from Fiction in Nutritional Science

In the world of nutrition, myths and misconceptions abound, making it challenging to navigate the sea of information surrounding dieting and healthy eating. It is essential to separate fact from fiction and rely on evidence-based practices to make informed food choices. Some common myths and realities of dieting include:

- **Myth**: Carbs are bad for you: In reality, carbohydrates are an essential source of energy and play a crucial role in a balanced diet. Opting for whole grains, fruits, and vegetables can provide valuable nutrients and fiber.

- **Myth: All fats are unhealthy**: While saturated and trans fats should be limited, healthy fats such as those found in avocados, nuts, and olive oil are beneficial for heart health and overall well-being.

- **Myth: You need to follow a strict diet to be healthy**: In reality, a balanced and varied diet that includes a wide range of foods can provide all the nutrients your body needs for optimal health.

By debunking these myths and embracing evidence-based nutritional practices, individuals can make informed food choices, support healthy aging, and promote longevity through a balanced and sustainable approach to eating well.

Chapter 5: Physical Activity and Aging

Regular physical activity is crucial for maintaining overall health and well-being, especially as we age. In this chapter, we will explore the importance of exercise in combating the aging process, how to tailor fitness routines to build strength and flexibility at different ages, and the benefits of practices like yoga and Tai Chi for holistic health.

Exercise as Medicine
Physical activity is often referred to as "exercise medicine" because of its powerful effects on the body. Regular exercise can help prevent or manage a wide range of health conditions,

including heart disease, diabetes, and arthritis. As we age, our bodies naturally undergo changes that can lead to a decline in muscle mass, bone density, and overall physical function. However, engaging in regular physical activity can help slow down these age-related changes and improve quality of life.

Building Strength and Flexibility
Strength training is essential for maintaining muscle mass and bone density, especially as we get older. By incorporating exercises that target different muscle groups, individuals can improve their strength, balance, and coordination. Flexibility exercises, such as stretching and yoga, can help maintain joint mobility and prevent injuries. It's important to tailor fitness routines to individual needs and abilities, taking into account factors like age, fitness level, and any existing health conditions.

The Mind-Body Connection
In addition to physical benefits, exercise also has profound effects on mental and emotional well-being. Practices like yoga, Tai Chi, and meditation emphasize the mind-body connection, promoting relaxation, stress reduction, and improved mental clarity. These holistic approaches to health can help older adults manage symptoms of anxiety, depression, and cognitive decline. By incorporating mind-body practices into their fitness routines, individuals can experience a greater sense of overall well-being.

Benefits of Cardiovascular Exercise
Cardiovascular exercise, such as walking, cycling, or swimming, is essential for maintaining heart health and overall fitness. Regular aerobic activity can help improve circulation, lower blood pressure, and reduce the risk of chronic diseases. For older adults, low-impact cardio exercises are ideal for improving cardiovascular endurance without

putting too much strain on the joints. By incorporating cardio workouts into their fitness routines, individuals can boost their energy levels and enhance their overall quality of life.

Nutrition and Physical Activity
A balanced diet plays a crucial role in supporting physical activity and overall health. Proper nutrition provides the fuel needed for exercise, helping to optimize performance and recovery. As we age, our nutritional needs may change, requiring adjustments to ensure adequate intake of essential nutrients. By following a well-rounded diet that includes a variety of fruits, vegetables, whole grains, and lean proteins, individuals can support their fitness goals and promote longevity.

Overcoming Barriers to Exercise
While the benefits of physical activity are clear, many older adults face barriers to staying active. Common obstacles include limited mobility, chronic pain, and lack of motivation. By

addressing these barriers through adaptive exercise programs, social support, and goal setting, individuals can overcome challenges and establish sustainable fitness habits. It's important to find activities that are enjoyable and engaging, making it easier to stay committed to a regular exercise routine.

Incorporating Functional Fitness
Functional fitness focuses on exercises that mimic everyday movements, helping individuals maintain strength and flexibility for daily activities. By incorporating functional exercises like squats, lunges, and core workouts, older adults can improve their balance, coordination, and overall physical function. These practical exercises are designed to enhance mobility and prevent falls, supporting independent living and a higher quality of life.

Staying Active in Older Age
As we age, it's important to prioritize physical activity as a key component of healthy aging. By

staying active through regular exercise, older adults can maintain their independence, vitality, and overall well-being. Whether it's taking daily walks, attending group fitness classes, or practicing yoga at home, finding activities that bring joy and fulfillment is essential for long-term health. With a proactive approach to fitness and aging, individuals can enjoy a higher quality of life and age gracefully.

The Role of Physical Therapy
Physical therapy plays a vital role in helping older adults recover from injuries, manage chronic conditions, and improve physical function. Through personalized treatment plans and targeted exercises, physical therapists can help individuals regain strength, mobility, and flexibility. Whether recovering from surgery or seeking relief from chronic pain, physical therapy can provide valuable support in restoring and maintaining optimal physical health.

Community Resources for Active Aging
Community resources play a key role in promoting active aging and supporting older adults in their fitness goals. Senior centers, fitness classes, and recreational programs offer opportunities for social engagement, physical activity, and learning. By connecting with local resources and participating in group activities, older adults can stay motivated, connected, and healthy. These community-based programs provide a supportive environment for individuals to pursue their fitness goals and enjoy an active lifestyle.

Technology and Fitness for Older Adults
Advancements in technology have made it easier than ever for older adults to stay active and engaged in their fitness routines. Fitness trackers, exercise apps, and online workout videos provide convenient tools for monitoring progress, setting goals, and accessing guided workouts. Virtual fitness classes and telehealth services offer flexibility and accessibility,

allowing individuals to stay connected with fitness professionals and healthcare providers from the comfort of their homes. By embracing technology, older adults can enhance their fitness experience and stay motivated to achieve their health and wellness goals.

Creating a Personalized Fitness Plan
When it comes to physical activity and aging, there is no one-size-fits-all approach. It's important to create a personalized fitness plan that takes into account individual goals, preferences, and limitations. Consulting with a fitness professional or healthcare provider can help tailor a workout routine that is safe, effective, and enjoyable. By setting realistic goals, tracking progress, and making adjustments as needed, individuals can stay motivated and committed to their fitness journey. Remember, it's never too late to start reaping the benefits of regular physical activity and embracing a healthier, more active lifestyle.

In conclusion, physical activity plays a vital role in promoting healthy aging and overall well-being. By incorporating regular exercise, strength training, and mind-body practices into daily routines, older adults can maintain their physical function, mental clarity, and emotional balance. With a proactive approach to fitness and a commitment to staying active, individuals can enjoy a higher quality of life and age gracefully. Remember, it's never too late to prioritize your health and well-being through physical activity. Start today and reap the countless benefits of staying active as you age.

Chapter 6: Technological Advances in Aging

In this chapter, we will delve into the exciting world of technological advances in aging, exploring recent breakthroughs in anti-aging research, predicting the future of medicine in longevity science, and navigating the ethical considerations surrounding extending life. From cutting-edge discoveries to ethical dilemmas, the intersection of technology and aging offers a glimpse into a future where living longer, healthier lives is not just a dream but a reality.

The Cutting Edge: Recent Breakthroughs in Anti-Aging Research

Recent years have seen remarkable advancements in anti-aging research, with scientists uncovering new ways to slow down the aging process and promote longevity. One groundbreaking discovery is the role of telomeres in cellular aging. Telomeres are protective caps at the end of chromosomes that shorten with each cell division, eventually leading to cell death. Researchers have found that telomere-lengthening therapies, such as telomerase activation, can potentially reverse cellular aging and extend lifespan.

Another exciting breakthrough is the development of senolytics, compounds that target and eliminate senescent cells, which are cells that have stopped dividing and accumulate with age. By clearing out these "zombie cells," senolytics have shown promise in delaying age-related diseases and extending their health span. Additionally, research on caloric restriction mimetics, such as resveratrol and metformin, has revealed their potential to mimic the effects of calorie restriction, a well-known longevity intervention.

Furthermore, advancements in regenerative medicine, including stem cell therapy and tissue engineering, hold great promise for rejuvenating aging tissues and organs. Stem cells have the unique ability to differentiate into various cell types, offering potential treatments for age-related conditions like osteoarthritis and neurodegenerative diseases. Tissue engineering techniques, such as 3D bioprinting, enable the creation of personalized implants and organs, revolutionizing the field of regenerative medicine.

Each of these discoveries has the potential to positively impact aging by slowing down the biological clock, enhancing cellular repair mechanisms, and promoting overall health and vitality. By harnessing the power of these cutting-edge technologies, researchers are paving the way for a future where age-related diseases are not just treated but prevented, and where individuals can enjoy extended years of healthy, active living.

The Future of Medicine: Predicting the Next Big Discoveries in Longevity Science
As we look ahead to the future of medicine and longevity science, several key areas are poised to drive significant advancements in aging research. One promising avenue is personalized medicine, which tailors treatments to individual genetic profiles, lifestyle factors, and health goals. By leveraging technologies like genomics, proteomics, and artificial intelligence, researchers can identify personalized interventions that optimize healthspan and lifespan.

Another frontier in longevity science is the microbiome, the diverse community of microorganisms that inhabit the human body. Emerging research suggests that the gut microbiome plays a crucial role in aging and age-related diseases, influencing metabolism, immune function, and inflammation. Manipulating the microbiome through probiotics, prebiotics, and fecal transplants holds the potential for modulating aging processes and promoting healthy aging.

Furthermore, the field of epigenetics, which studies how gene expression is regulated by environmental factors, offers insights into the molecular mechanisms of aging. Epigenetic modifications, such as DNA methylation and histone acetylation, can be influenced by lifestyle choices, stress, and environmental exposures. Understanding how epigenetic changes impact aging could lead to targeted interventions that slow down the aging process and prevent age-related diseases.

Additionally, advancements in artificial intelligence and machine learning are revolutionizing healthcare by analyzing vast amounts of data to predict disease risk, optimize treatment strategies, and improve patient outcomes. AI-powered diagnostics, predictive modeling, and drug discovery platforms are transforming the way we approach aging-related conditions, offering personalized solutions that enhance quality of life and longevity.

By staying at the forefront of these cutting-edge technologies and research trends, the future of medicine holds immense promise for extending healthy lifespans, preventing age-related diseases, and enhancing overall well-being. As scientists continue to unravel the complexities of aging and develop innovative interventions, the possibilities for living longer, healthier lives are becoming increasingly within reach.

Ethics and Aging: Navigating the Moral Implications of Extending Life
While the advancements in anti-aging research and longevity science offer tremendous potential for improving health and longevity, they also raise important ethical considerations that must

be carefully navigated. One of the key ethical dilemmas is the concept of **"healthspan extension,"** which focuses on extending the period of healthy, active life rather than simply prolonging lifespan. By prioritizing healthspan, individuals can enjoy more years of vitality and independence, free from age-related disabilities and chronic conditions.

Another ethical issue is the equitable distribution of anti-aging interventions and technologies. As breakthroughs in aging research become available, ensuring equal access to these treatments for individuals of all socioeconomic backgrounds is essential. Addressing disparities in healthcare access and affordability is crucial for promoting health equity and social justice in the context of aging populations.

Furthermore, the concept of **"radical life extension,"** or significantly prolonging human lifespan beyond current limits, raises questions about the implications for society, the environment, and individual well-being. Ethical considerations around resource allocation, population growth, and existential questions about the nature of life and death come to the forefront when discussing radical life extension technologies.

Moreover, issues of autonomy, informed consent, and privacy must be carefully considered in the development and implementation of anti-aging interventions. Individuals should have the right to make informed decisions about their health and well-being, including whether to pursue anti-aging treatments and technologies. Respecting individual autonomy and ensuring transparency in the use of personal health data are essential ethical principles in the field of aging research.

As we navigate the complex ethical landscape of extending life through technological advances, it is crucial to engage in thoughtful dialogue, ethical reflection, and interdisciplinary collaboration. By addressing these ethical considerations with compassion, empathy, and foresight, we can ensure that advancements in aging research are guided by principles of beneficence, justice, and respect for human dignity.

In conclusion, technological advances in aging hold immense promise for transforming the landscape of health and longevity. From cutting-edge discoveries in anti-aging research to the future of medicine in longevity science, and the ethical considerations surrounding extending life, the intersection of technology and aging offers a glimpse into a future where aging is not just a biological process but a modifiable one. By harnessing the power of innovative technologies, personalized interventions, and ethical frameworks, we can pave the way for a future where individuals can age with grace, vitality, and dignity. As we continue to explore the frontiers of anti-aging research and longevity science, let us embrace the possibilities of living longer, healthier lives and strive to create a world where aging is not a barrier but an opportunity for growth, resilience, and well-being. Together, we can shape a future where age is just a number, and the journey of aging is one filled with vitality, purpose, and joy.

Chapter 7: Personal Stories of Longevity

In this chapter, we will explore personal stories of longevity, highlighting individuals who defy the aging process, sharing secrets and insights from centenarians, and showcasing inspirational tales of resilience and health. Through the lens of personal narratives, we gain a deeper understanding of the factors that contribute to

living a long, healthy life. Let's begin with the story of Mr. Oliver Dowen, a remarkable individual who has lived 95 years and embodies the principles of prioritizing health and well-being throughout his life.

Mr. Oliver Dowen: A Lifetime of Prioritizing Health

Mr. Oliver Dowen, a sprightly 95-year-old gentleman, has always been passionate about taking care of his health. From a young age, Oliver showed a keen interest in learning about nutrition, exercise, and overall well-being. As a boy, he would spend hours reading books on health and wellness, absorbing knowledge like a sponge. This early curiosity laid the foundation for a lifetime of dedication to maintaining his health.

In his 20s, Oliver cultivated the habit of regular exercise, incorporating activities like walking, swimming, and gardening into his daily routine.

He understood the importance of staying active to keep his body strong and agile. As he entered his 30s and 40s, Oliver made conscious choices to adjust his diet, focusing on whole foods, fruits, vegetables, and lean proteins. He avoided eating late at night, opting for lighter meals that were easy to digest.

One of the key habits that Oliver adopted early on was scheduling regular medical checkups. By staying proactive about his health, Oliver was able to catch any potential issues early and address them promptly. Whether it was a routine physical exam or a consultation with a specialist, Oliver made sure to prioritize his health and well-being above all else.

As the years passed, Oliver continued to make adjustments to his lifestyle, listening to his body and making changes where necessary. He understood the importance of balance, moderation, and consistency in maintaining his health. By staying disciplined, focused, and

proactive, Oliver was able to age gracefully and enjoy a high quality of life well into his golden years.

Living Legends: Secrets and Insights on Longevity

1. Stay Active: Many living legends attribute their longevity to staying physically active throughout their lives. Engaging in regular exercise, whether it's walking, dancing, or yoga, helps maintain muscle strength, flexibility, and overall vitality.

2. Eat Well: A healthy diet rich in fruits, vegetables, whole grains, and lean proteins is a common theme among centenarians. Eating a balanced diet provides essential nutrients that support overall health and well-being.

3. Stay Social: Building strong social connections and maintaining relationships with friends and family contribute to emotional well-being and longevity. Social interaction provides a sense of belonging and purpose.

4. Stay Curious: Lifelong learning and intellectual stimulation are key factors in staying sharp and engaged as we age. Reading, learning new skills, and staying curious about the world around us keep the mind active and vibrant.

5. Practice Gratitude: Expressing gratitude and maintaining a positive outlook on life have been linked to better health outcomes and increased longevity. Cultivating a sense of gratitude for the present moment fosters emotional resilience and well-being.

6. Embrace Change: Flexibility and adaptability are essential traits for living a long, fulfilling life. Embracing change, learning from challenges, and staying open to new experiences promote growth and resilience.

Overcoming Challenges: Inspirational Tales of Resilience and Health

In the realm of longevity and well-being, there are countless stories of individuals who have overcome significant challenges with resilience, determination, and a commitment to their health. These inspirational tales serve as reminders of the human spirit's capacity to triumph over adversity and emerge stronger, healthier, and more vibrant. Let's explore some of these remarkable stories that showcase the power of resilience and health in the face of challenges.

1. The Story of Maria Santos: A Journey of Healing and Strength

Maria Santos, a 70-year-old grandmother, faced a daunting health challenge when she was diagnosed with a chronic autoimmune condition that left her fatigued, in pain, and struggling to perform daily tasks. Despite the physical and emotional toll of her illness, Maria refused to let

it define her. With the support of her family and healthcare team, Maria embarked on a journey of healing and strength.

Through a combination of medical treatment, lifestyle changes, and a positive mindset, Maria gradually regained her health and vitality. She embraced holistic approaches to wellness, incorporating meditation, yoga, and nutritious eating into her daily routine. By prioritizing self-care and listening to her body's needs, Maria was able to overcome her health challenges and emerge stronger than ever.

Maria's story is a testament to the power of resilience, perseverance, and the human body's remarkable ability to heal. By staying committed to her health and well-being, Maria not only conquered her illness but also inspired those around her to prioritize self-care and resilience in the face of adversity.

2. The Journey of John Parker: From Setback to Comeback

John Parker, a 60-year-old retiree, faced a major setback when he suffered a heart attack that left him physically weak and emotionally shaken. Determined to reclaim his health and vitality, John embarked on a journey of recovery and renewal. With the guidance of his healthcare team and the unwavering support of his loved ones, John committed to making positive changes to his lifestyle and habits.

Through cardiac rehabilitation, regular exercise, and a heart-healthy diet, John gradually regained his strength and confidence. He embraced new opportunities for physical activity, such as swimming and cycling, that not only improved his cardiovascular health but also boosted his mood and overall well-being. By staying resilient in the face of adversity, John transformed his setback into a comeback, proving that with determination and perseverance, anything is possible.

John's journey serves as a reminder that challenges can be overcome with resilience, support, and a proactive approach to health. By taking ownership of his well-being and making positive choices, John not only recovered from his heart attack but also embraced a new lease on life filled with vitality, purpose, and gratitude.

3. The Resilience of Sarah Chang: A Story of Strength and Hope

Sarah Chang, an 80-year-old cancer survivor, exemplifies the power of resilience, strength, and hope in the face of adversity. Diagnosed with breast cancer in her late 60s, Sarah faced a daunting treatment journey that tested her physical and emotional resilience. Despite the challenges of chemotherapy, surgery, and radiation, Sarah remained steadfast in her determination to overcome cancer and reclaim her health.

Through the unwavering support of her healthcare team, family, and friends, Sarah navigated the complexities of cancer treatment with grace and courage. She embraced complementary therapies, such as acupuncture and meditation, to support her healing journey and alleviate treatment side effects. By staying positive, hopeful, and proactive in her care, Sarah emerged from her cancer battle stronger, more resilient, and with a renewed appreciation for life.

Sarah's story is a testament to the resilience of the human spirit and the transformative power of hope in the face of adversity. By embodying strength, courage, and a positive mindset, Sarah not only conquered cancer but also inspired others to approach life's challenges with grace, resilience, and unwavering hope.

These inspirational tales of resilience and health remind us that challenges can be overcome with determination, support, and a commitment to prioritizing well-being. By drawing strength from these stories of triumph over adversity, we are inspired to embrace our health journeys with resilience, courage, and a belief in the power of the human spirit to overcome obstacles and emerge stronger, healthier, and more vibrant.

Conclusion

As we reach the end of this book on aging, longevity, and well-being, it is time to reflect on the transformative journey we have embarked on together. From exploring the latest technological advances in anti-aging research to delving into personal stories of resilience and health, we have uncovered a wealth of insights, inspiration, and wisdom that illuminate the path to living a long, healthy, and fulfilling life. Let us take a moment to integrate the science and emotion that have guided us through this exploration and envision a future where longevity is not just a dream but a reality.

Integrating Science and Emotion: A Reflection on the Journey Through the Book

Throughout this book, we have witnessed the powerful intersection of science and emotion in shaping our understanding of aging and well-being. From the cutting-edge discoveries in anti-aging research to the inspirational tales of resilience and health, we have seen how a holistic approach to health encompasses not only physical well-being but also emotional resilience, mental clarity, and spiritual vitality. By integrating the latest scientific advancements with the human experience of aging, we have gained a deeper appreciation for the multifaceted nature of longevity and the importance of nurturing both body and soul as we journey through life.

The Path Forward: How Readers Can Apply the Book's Insights to Their Own Lives
As readers, you now hold a treasure trove of insights, strategies, and inspiration to guide you on your path to healthy aging and well-being. From prioritizing physical activity and nutrition to cultivating resilience and embracing change,

the lessons learned from this book can serve as a roadmap for creating a life filled with vitality, purpose, and joy. By applying the principles of longevity science, personal stories of resilience, and living legends' secrets to your own life, you can embark on a transformative journey toward a healthier, happier, and more fulfilling future.

A Timeless Future: Envisioning a World Where Longevity is the Norm
As we look ahead to the future, let us envision a world where longevity is not just a privilege but a universal norm. By embracing the principles of healthy aging, prioritizing well-being, and fostering a culture of resilience and vitality, we can create a timeless future where individuals of all ages can thrive, flourish, and live their best lives. Through collective action, scientific innovation, and a shared commitment to promoting health and longevity, we can pave the way for a world where age is celebrated, wisdom is revered, and life is cherished in all its beauty and complexity.

In closing, may this book serve as a beacon of hope, inspiration, and empowerment as you

navigate your own journey through the intricacies of aging, well-being, and longevity. Remember, the path to a long, healthy, and fulfilling life begins with a single step, a commitment to self-care, and a belief in the infinite possibilities that each day brings. Embrace the wisdom gained from these pages, carry it forward with grace and gratitude, and embark on a timeless journey towards a future where age is but a number, and the essence of life is eternal.

IF YOU GOT VALUE FROM THIS BOOK, KINDLY LEAVE A REVIEW FOR ME ONLINE. THANK YOU

YOU CAN CHECK MY OTHER BOOKS HERE
https://www.amazon.com/author/elvygraves

www.ingramcontent.com/pod-product-compliance
Lightning Source LLC
Chambersburg PA
CBHW050236230526
45470CB00005B/1976